Excellence In Medicine

Mbuso Mabuza

Published by Mbuso Mabuza, 2026.

EXCELLENCE IN MEDICINE

First edition. February 11, 2026.

ISBN: 979-8233988820

Written by Mbuso Mabuza.

Also by Mbuso Mabuza

A Healthy Mind And Best You: Achieving Great Results in Every Aspect of Your Life
Purposeful And Better You
Efficacy, Effectiveness And Efficiency In The Management Of Health Systems
Promoting Health and Wellbeing
Medicine and the Sociology of Health
Qualitative Methods In Public Health Research
Global Health Disaster Management
Global Health Policy And Programme Challenges
The Journey of Life Has a Gift of Purpose
Epidemiological Research
Ethics, Qualitative And Quantitative Methods In Public Health Research
Emotional Intelligence in Relationships
Blockchain Technology In Healthcare And Medicine
Immersive Technologies In Healthcare: Virtual Reality And Augmented Reality
Health Data Analytics And Informatics
How To Improve The Way You Think
Health Systems Engineering: Building A Better Healthcare Delivery System
Artificial Intelligence In Drug Discovery And Development
How To Make The Most Of Life
Precision Medicine

Connected Health: Technology-Enabled Care
Person Centered Care And Optimal Wellbeing
Reimagine Your Tomorrow
Leading Remote Teams in the 21st Century
Qualitative Research In Health and Medicine
Excellence In Medicine

Table of Contents

To the healers of today and the leaders of tomorrow: May this guide serve as a steady companion in your pursuit of clinical mastery. This work is dedicated to those who recognize that the greatest medicine is a blend of scientific excellence, unwavering ethics, and the simple, profound act of listening.

"In the face of uncertainty, the clinician's greatest tools are not just the stethoscope and the scalpel, but a disciplined mind, an ethical heart, and the courage to remain human." — **Anonymous**

Introduction

Excellence in Medicine: A Practical Guide to Clinical Mastery, Ethical Practice, and Patient-Cantered Care is designed as a comprehensive resource for medical professionals at all stages of their careers, from medical students to seasoned practitioners. This book addresses the multifaceted nature of medical excellence, moving beyond mere technical competence to encompass ethical considerations, effective communication, cultural sensitivity, and a commitment to lifelong learning.

In an era of rapidly evolving medical knowledge, technological advancements, and increasing healthcare complexity, the pursuit of excellence is not merely an aspiration but a necessity. Patients deserve nothing less than the best possible care, delivered with compassion, integrity, and a dedication to continuous improvement. This book aims to provide a roadmap for achieving and sustaining such excellence in all aspects of medical practice.

The motivation behind this book stems from a recognition that traditional medical education, while strong in imparting scientific knowledge, often falls short in preparing clinicians for the real-world challenges of practice. The pressures of demanding schedules, complex patient cases, and the ever-present threat of litigation can erode even the most well-intentioned physician's commitment to excellence. Furthermore, the increasing emphasis on efficiency and cost-effectiveness can sometimes overshadow the importance of patient-centred care and ethical considerations.

This book seeks to bridge this gap by providing practical guidance on a wide range of topics, including:

Clinical Reasoning

Developing the critical thinking skills necessary to accurately diagnose and manage complex medical conditions. We will explore cognitive biases, diagnostic heuristics, and strategies for avoiding common errors in clinical judgment.

(Croskerry, P. (2003). Cognitive forcing strategies in clinical decision making. Annals of Emergency Medicine, 42(1), 110-120.)

Evidence-Based Medicine

Integrating the best available research evidence with clinical expertise and patient values to make informed treatment decisions. We will discuss how to critically appraise research studies, interpret statistical data, and apply evidence to individual patient cases.

(Sackett, D. L., et al. (2000). Evidence-based medicine: How to practice and teach EBM. Churchill Livingstone.)

Ethical Practice

Navigating the complex ethical dilemmas that arise in modern medicine, such as end-of-life care, informed consent, and resource allocation. We will examine ethical frameworks, case studies, and strategies for resolving ethical conflicts.

(Beauchamp, T. L., & Childress, J. F. (2019). Principles of biomedical ethics (8th ed.). Oxford University Press.)

Communication Skills

Mastering the art of effective communication with patients, families, and colleagues. We will explore techniques for active listening, empathy, and shared decision-making.

(Epstein, R. M., & Street, R. L., Jr. (2007). Patient-centered communication in cancer care: Promoting healing and hope. National Cancer Institute.)

Cultural Competence

Providing culturally sensitive care to patients from diverse backgrounds. We will discuss the importance of understanding cultural beliefs, values, and practices, and how to adapt our communication and treatment approaches accordingly.

(Betancourt, J. R., et al. (2003). Defining cultural competence: a practical framework... Public Health Reports, 118(4), 293.)

Quality Improvement and Patient Safety

Implementing strategies to improve the quality and safety of medical care. We will explore methodologies such as Lean, Six Sigma, and root cause analysis, and discuss how to create a culture of safety.

(Berwick, D. M. (2003). Improvement as a science. Annals of Internal Medicine, 138(11), 903-908.)

Well-being and Resilience

Addressing the challenges of burnout and promoting well-being in medical practice. We will discuss strategies for managing stress, improving work-life balance, and fostering a sense of purpose and meaning.

(Shanafelt, T. D., et al. (2012). Burnout and satisfaction with work-life balance among US physicians... Archives of Internal Medicine, 172(18), 1377-1385.)

This book is not intended to be a theoretical treatise but rather a practical guide, filled with real-world examples, case studies, and actionable strategies. Each chapter will include learning objectives, key concepts, self-assessment questions, and recommended resources for further study.

As you journey through these chapters, I invite you to reflect on your own practice, challenge your assumptions, and embrace the ongoing process of professional growth. Excellence is not a destination but a continuous path of refinement—one where scientific rigor meets humanistic care.

Ultimately, our goal is to inspire a new generation of medical professionals who are not only technically competent but also compassionate, ethical, and committed to lifelong learning. I believe that by embracing these principles, we can create a healthcare system that is truly patient-centred, equitable, and sustainable.

Sincerely,

Dr. Mbuso Mabuza

Chapter 1: The Foundation of Excellence: Defining Competence and Beyond

Learning Objectives

- After studying this chapter, you should be able to:
- Define medical competence and distinguish it from medical excellence.
- Identify and describe the six core competencies established by the ACGME.
- Explain the role of education, residency, and continuous training in developing professional mastery.
- Discuss the key elements that elevate a physician's practice from basic competence to true excellence.
- Analyse real-world examples of patient-centred care and institutional excellence.

Introduction

The pursuit of excellence in medicine begins with a solid foundation of competence. Competence, in its most basic form, refers to the possession of the requisite knowledge, skills, and attitudes necessary to perform a specific task or role effectively. In medicine, this translates to the ability to accurately diagnose and treat medical conditions, communicate effectively with patients and colleagues, and adhere to ethical and legal standards of practice.

However, excellence extends far beyond mere competence. It encompasses a commitment to continuous improvement, a dedication to patient-centred care, and a passion for lifelong learning. This chapter will explore the concept of competence in medicine, examine the factors that contribute to its development, and discuss how to move beyond competence to achieve true excellence.

Defining Competence in Medicine

Medical competence is a complex and multifaceted construct, encompassing a range of cognitive, psychomotor, and affective skills. The Accreditation Council for Graduate Medical Education (ACGME) has identified six core competencies that are essential for all physicians:

Patient Care: The ability to provide compassionate, appropriate, and effective care. This includes skills in history taking, physical examination, diagnosis, treatment planning, and patient education.

Medical Knowledge: The possession of a comprehensive and up-to-date understanding of biomedical, clinical, and social sciences.

Practice-Based Learning and Improvement: The ability to critically evaluate one's own performance and implement strategies to enhance one's practice.

Interpersonal and Communication Skills: The ability to communicate effectively and sensitively with patients, families, and other healthcare professionals.

Professionalism: The demonstration of a commitment to ethical principles, integrity, and sensitivity to a diverse patient population.

Systems-Based Practice: The ability to understand and navigate the healthcare system, including its organizational structure and regulatory requirements.

These six core competencies provide a framework for assessing and developing competence in medical practice. However, it is important to recognize that competence is not a static state but rather a dynamic process that requires continuous effort and refinement.

Developing Competence: Education, Training, and Experience

The development of competence in medicine is a lifelong journey that begins with formal medical education and continues through residency training, fellowship programs, and continuing medical education. Each stage of this journey plays a crucial role in shaping the knowledge, skills, and attitudes of future physicians.

Medical Education: Provides the foundational knowledge and skills through basic and clinical sciences.

Residency Training: A period of intensive clinical experience under supervision, allowing for the refinement of diagnostic abilities.

Fellowship Programs: Provide advanced training in a specific medical subspecialty, fostering expertise and leadership.

Continuing Medical Education (CME): An ongoing process essential for maintaining competence and staying updated on medical advances.

In addition to formal education, experience plays a critical role. As physicians gain experience, they develop a deeper understanding of disease processes and refine their clinical judgment. Experience also helps in developing the interpersonal skills necessary to build trust and rapport with patients.

Moving Beyond Competence: The Pursuit of Excellence

While competence is essential for safe and effective medical practice, it is not sufficient for achieving true excellence. Excellence in medicine requires a commitment to continuous improvement, a dedication to patient-centred care, and a passion for lifelong learning.

Key Elements of Excellence:

Patient-Cantered Care: Excellent physicians prioritize the needs and preferences of their patients, building therapeutic relationships and empowering them.

Ethical Practice: Adhering to the highest ethical standards, even when making difficult decisions in complex situations.

Continuous Improvement: Constantly seeking ways to improve and actively seeking feedback from colleagues and patients.

Lifelong Learning: Cultivating a habit of curiosity and a desire to learn from every patient encounter.

Leadership: Inspiring and empowering others, setting an example, and advocating for positive change within the healthcare system.

Case Study: Dr. Emily Carter

Dr. Emily Carter is a cardiologist at a large academic medical centre. She is widely regarded as an excellent physician by her colleagues and patients alike. Dr. Carter is known for her exceptional clinical skills, her compassionate approach to patient care, and her unwavering commitment to ethical practice. Dr. Carter is a strong advocate for patient-centred care. She always takes the time to listen to her patients and involve them in decision making. As a leader in her field, she mentors medical students and advocates for patient safety and quality improvement.

Real-World Example: The Mayo Clinic

The Mayo Clinic is widely regarded as one of the best healthcare organizations in the world. It is known for its commitment to patient-centred care, integrated team-based clinical practice, and its motto: "The needs of the patient come first." Their culture of collaboration among physicians, nurses, and researchers serves as a global benchmark for medical excellence.

Conclusion

Excellence in medicine is a journey, not a destination. It requires a commitment to continuous improvement, a dedication to patient-centred care, and a passion for lifelong learning. By embracing these principles, medical professionals can provide the best possible care to their patients and make a positive impact on the world. While competence is the bedrock, the pursuit of excellence elevates the practice of medicine to its highest potential.

References

Accreditation Council for Graduate Medical Education (ACGME). (2023). ACGME common program requirements.

Berwick, D. M. (2003). Improvement as a science. Annals of Internal Medicine, 138(11), 903-908.

Mann, K. V. (2011). Self-regulated learning strategies for lifelong learning. Medical Education, 45(5), 444-454.

Maxwell, J. C. (2007). The 21 irrefutable laws of leadership: Follow them and people will follow you. Thomas Nelson Inc.

Mead, N., & Bower, P. (2000). Patient-centredness: a conceptual framework and review of the empirical literature. Social Science & Medicine, 51(7), 1087-1110.

Pellegrino, E. D., & Thomasma, D. C. (1993). The virtues in medical practice. Oxford University Press.

Chapter 2: Mastering the Art of Diagnosis: Clinical Reasoning and Differential Diagnosis

Learning Objectives

- By the end of this chapter, the reader will be able to:
- Outline the five iterative steps of the diagnostic clinical reasoning framework.
- Identify and define common cognitive biases, including availability heuristic, confirmation bias, anchoring, and premature closure.
- Apply the VINDICATE+ mnemonic to generate a comprehensive differential diagnosis.
- Utilize metacognitive strategies and 'diagnostic time-outs' to improve diagnostic accuracy.
- Discuss the evolving role of AI as a 'diagnostic co-pilot' in the clinical setting.

Introduction

Accurate and timely diagnosis is the cornerstone of effective medical care. The diagnostic process involves a complex interplay of clinical reasoning, pattern recognition, and hypothesis testing. Mastering the art of diagnosis requires a deep understanding of disease pathophysiology, a keen ability to elicit and interpret clinical data, and a systematic approach to differential diagnosis. This chapter will explore the principles of clinical reasoning, discuss common cognitive biases that can affect diagnostic accuracy, and provide practical strategies for developing a robust differential diagnosis.

The Diagnostic Process: A Framework for Clinical Reasoning

The diagnostic process can be conceptualized as a series of iterative steps:

- Data Acquisition: Gathering relevant information (history, physical, labs, imaging).
- Problem Representation: Synthesizing data into a coherent clinical narrative.
- Hypothesis Generation: Creating a list of common and rare possibilities.
- Hypothesis Evaluation: Considering pre-test probability and evidence.
- Diagnosis Verification: Confirming via biopsy, testing, or treatment response.
- Cognitive Biases in Diagnosis: Avoiding Common Pitfalls

Cognitive biases are systematic errors in thinking. Common biases include:

- Availability Heuristic: Overestimating likely events based on recent memory.
- Confirmation Bias: Seeking info that confirms existing beliefs.
- Anchoring Bias: Relying too heavily on initial information.
- Premature Closure: Stopping the search once a plausible answer is found.

Developing a Robust Differential Diagnosis

To ensure comprehensive coverage, clinicians should utilize the following strategies:

Consider Patient Demographics: Accounts for age, gender, race, and ancestry.

Utilize Mnemonics: The VINDICATE+ mnemonic ensures all categories of disease are considered:

V - Vascular
I - Infectious/Inflammatory
N - Neoplastic
D - Degenerative/Deficiency/Drugs
I - Idiopathic/Iatrogenic/Intoxication
C - Congenital
A - Autoimmune/Allergic
T - Traumatic
E - Endocrine/Metabolic

Assess Probabilities: Rank the list into 'Must-not-miss' (life-threatening), 'Leading hypothesis' (most likely), and 'Alternatives.'

CASE STUDY: THE DANGER OF PREMATURE CLOSURE

Clinical Case: A 52-year-old male presents with sharp chest pain and shortness of breath. The clinician 'anchors' on Acute Coronary Syndrome (ACS) based on history and EKG.

The Pitfall: After 4 hours, the pain shifts to his back and blood pressure fluctuates between arms. A CT angiogram finally reveals an Aortic Dissection.

Reflection: "The eyes do not see what the mind does not look for."

Metacognition: Thinking About Thinking

Metacognition involves 'diagnostic time-outs' to evaluate one's own thought processes. Strategies include using de-biasing checklists, seeking second opinions, and simulation-based training.

The Evolution of Diagnostic Mastery

Expertise is characterized by the transition from rote algorithmic thinking to sophisticated pattern recognition. Recent studies highlight the use of Artificial Intelligence (AI) as a 'diagnostic co-pilot,' where the 'human-in-the-loop' model yields the highest accuracy.

Conclusion

Excellence in medicine begins with the humility to realize that every diagnosis is a hypothesis waiting to be tested. By maintaining a disciplined approach, the physician fulfils their primary duty: to see the patient truly and clearly.

REFERENCES

Croskerry, P. (2003). The Importance of Cognitive Errors in Diagnosis and Strategies to Minimize Them. Academic Medicine, 78(8), 775-780.

Groopman, J. (2007). How Doctors Think. Houghton Mifflin Harcourt.

Grosse, S. D., et al. (2004). Newborn Screening for Cystic Fibrosis: Evaluation of Benefits and Risks. MMWR Recommendations and Reports, 53(RR-13), 1-36.

Obermeyer, Z., & Emanuel, E. J. (2016). Predicting the Future — Big Data, Machine Learning, and Clinical Medicine. NEJM, 375(13), 1216-1219.

Chapter 3: Evidence-Based Medicine: Integrating Research into Clinical Practice

LEARNING OBJECTIVES

- After studying this chapter, you should be able to:
- Define Evidence-Based Medicine (EBM) and its role in clinical mastery.
- Apply the PICO framework to formulate answerable clinical questions.
- Identify and navigate the Hierarchy of Evidence to find the best clinical data.
- Appraise research for internal validity and clinical significance.
- Integrate scientific evidence with clinical expertise and patient values in practice.

"Medicine is a science of uncertainty and an art of probability." — Sir William Osler.

In the pursuit of clinical excellence, the practitioner must bridge the gap between burgeoning scientific discovery and the bedside. Evidence-Based Medicine (EBM) is not merely a formulaic application of research; it is the conscientious, explicit, and judicious use of current best evidence in making decisions about the care of individual patients (Sackett et al., 1996). Dr. Mbuso Mabuza posits that true clinical mastery requires an equilibrium. Relying solely on clinical 'gut feeling' without evidence is dangerous, yet relying solely on data without clinical context is mechanical. EBM serves as the framework for this equilibrium. It demands that the physician remains a lifelong student, acknowledging that today's gold standard may be tomorrow's obsolete practice. The integration of individual clinical expertise—defined as the proficiency and judgment acquired through clinical experience—is what allows a practitioner to determine if a trial's results apply to the unique human being sitting in the exam room (Guyatt et al., 2015).

The Five Essential Pillars of Practice

The practice of EBM is a dynamic, five-step cyclical process:

Asking the Answerable Question (PICO): Mastery begins with clarity. Using the PICO framework (Patient/Population, Intervention, Comparison, Outcome), a vague concern like "Should I use this drug?" becomes "In elderly patients with Type 2 Diabetes (P), does Metformin (I) compared to SGLT2 inhibitors (C) more effectively reduce cardiovascular mortality (O)?" (Richardson et al., 1995).

Acquiring the Evidence: In the digital age, the challenge is no longer finding information but filtering it. Practitioners must navigate databases like PubMed, Cochrane Library, and Embase with precision.

Appraising the Evidence: Not all published research is truth. Critical appraisal asks: Is the study valid (internal validity)? Is the effect size clinically significant? Are the results applicable to my patient?

Applying the Evidence: This is the 'Art of Medicine.' Here, the physician integrates the research with their own expertise and, crucially, the patient's unique values, preferences, and socio-economic context (Sackett et al., 2000).

Assessing Performance: This final stage is one of self-reflection. Did the application of this evidence lead to the desired outcome? How can the process be improved next time?

The Hierarchy of Evidence and Its Limitations

To navigate the sea of literature, we use the Evidence Pyramid. At the apex sit Systematic Reviews and Meta-analyses... (text abbreviated for brevity in code, but full text will be in doc).

To navigate the sea of literature, we use the Evidence Pyramid. At the apex sit Systematic Reviews and Meta-analyses, which synthesize multiple Randomized Controlled Trials (RCTs) to provide a high-level overview of a therapeutic's efficacy. Below these are individual RCTs, followed by Observational Studies (Cohort and Case-Control), and finally, Case Reports and Expert Opinion (Guyatt et al., 2008). However, Dr. Mabuza reminds us that the hierarchy is a guide, not a dogma. There are instances where RCTs are unethical or impossible—for example, measuring the efficacy of parachutes or the long-term effects of rare toxins. In such cases, high-quality observational data becomes our primary guide. The mastery lies in knowing when a lower level of evidence provides the highest level of practical utility. Reflective Thought: As you move up the pyramid, the risk of bias decreases, but the distance from the individual 'n-of-1' patient often increases. The clinician's role is to bring that data back down to the human scale.

Case Studies: EBM in Action

Case Study: The Balanced Anticoagulant Choice

Dr. Sarah Lin is treating Mr. Thompson, a 72-year-old with newly diagnosed Atrial Fibrillation. Traditional guidelines strongly suggest Warfarin. However, Dr. Lin performs a PICO search for Direct Oral Anticoagulants (DOACs) vs. Warfarin. She finds a meta-analysis indicating DOACs have a lower risk of intracranial haemorrhage (Granger et al., 2011). Integration: Mr. Thompson lives in a rural area and expresses a deep fear of frequent clinic visits for blood monitoring (INR). Despite the higher cost of DOACs, Dr. Lin and Mr. Thompson decide on Apixaban, aligning the best evidence (safety profile) with the patient's lifestyle values (preference for fewer tests).

Case Study: The Limitation of Expert Opinion

In the mid-20th century, it was "expert opinion" that infants should sleep on their stomachs to prevent choking. It wasn't until systematic reviews of observational data proved that prone sleeping was a major risk factor for SIDS (Sudden Infant Death Syndrome) that the "Back to Sleep" campaign began, saving thousands of lives (Gilbert et al., 2005). This serves as a humbling reminder to always question 'the way we've **always done it.'**

Conclusion

Excellence in medicine is a commitment to the truth, even when the truth is evolving. By embedding EBM into daily practice, Dr. Mbuso Mabuza encourages clinicians to move beyond 'eminence-based medicine' toward a practice that is verifiable, ethical, and profoundly patient-centred. Inspiration for the Practitioner: "The good physician treats the disease; the great physician treats the patient who has the disease." — William Osler.

References

Gilbert, R., et al. (2005). Infant sleeping position and the sudden infant death syndrome: systematic review of observational studies and historical review of recommendations from 1940 to 2002. International Journal of Epidemiology.

Granger, C. B., et al. (2011). Apixaban versus Warfarin in Patients with Atrial Fibrillation. New England Journal of Medicine.

Guyatt, G. H., et al. (2008). GRADE: an emerging consensus on rating quality of evidence and strength of recommendations. BMJ.

Guyatt, G. H., et al. (2015). Users' Guides to the Medical Literature: A Manual for Evidence-Based Clinical Practice. McGraw-Hill Education.

Richardson, W. S., et al. (1995). The well-built clinical question: a key to evidence-based decisions. ACP Journal Club.

Sackett, D. L., et al. (1996). Evidence based medicine: what it is and what it isn't. BMJ.

Sackett, D. L., et al. (2000). Evidence-Based Medicine: How to Practice and Teach EBM. Churchill Livingstone.

Chapter 4: The Therapeutic Alliance: Building Trust and Rapport with Patients

LEARNING OBJECTIVES

By the end of this chapter, students should be able to:

- Define the therapeutic alliance and its role in clinical outcomes.
- Contrast the historical paternalistic model with modern patient-physician dynamics.
- Apply the three-step model of Shared Decision-Making (SDM) in clinical scenarios.
- Identify the three pillars of the alliance according to Bordin's model.
- Analyse common barriers to rapport, including time constraints and technology.
- Demonstrate cultural humility and the application of 'Ubuntu' in global health settings.
- Utilize the 'SOLER' framework for effective non-verbal communication.

Introduction: The Heart of the Clinical Encounter

The relationship between a physician and a patient is the heart of medicine. Beyond the cold precision of diagnostic tests and pharmacological interventions lies a human connection that serves as the primary vehicle for healing. A strong therapeutic alliance is not merely a 'soft skill'; it is a clinical necessity associated with better treatment adherence, improved patient satisfaction, and superior clinical outcomes. It is the invisible force that transforms a clinical transaction into a healing journey.

"The good physician treats the disease; the great physician treats the patient who has the disease."

— *Sir William Osler*

The Evolution of the Patient-Physician Dynamic

Historically, medicine operated under a paternalistic model where the physician was the sole arbiter of truth, and the patient was a passive recipient of care. However, the modern clinical landscape demands a shift. The therapeutic alliance, a concept originally rooted in psychotherapy, has become central to all branches of medicine. It represents a shift toward a partnership characterized by mutual respect, shared goals, and emotional resonance. As noted by Balint (1957), 'the doctor is the most frequently used drug in general practice,' emphasizing the physician's own personality and presence as a therapeutic agent.

Empathy and Active Listening: The Gateway to Connection

Empathy is the ability to understand and share the feelings of another. In a clinical setting, this is not merely a feeling but a clinical competency. It involves active listening—giving the patient undivided attention and validating their experiences (Halpern, 2003). Active listening requires more than silence; it involves the 'clinical presence'—the ability to sit with a patient's pain without rushing to a diagnostic conclusion. Research has shown that physicians who demonstrate high levels of empathy are more likely to elicit critical diagnostic information from patients that might otherwise remain hidden due to shame or fear. Decety and Fotopoulou (2015) suggest that the neural mechanisms involved in empathy can modulate the patient's perception of pain, demonstrating a biological basis for the power of the alliance.

Shared Decision-Making: Beyond Consent

Moving away from paternalism, shared decision-making (SDM) involves a collaborative process where the clinician and patient reach a consensus on the best course of action, respecting the patient's autonomy and values (Charles et al., 1997). SDM is particularly crucial in 'preference-sensitive' conditions where there is no single 'correct' medical answer. The process follows a three-step model: Choice Talk (notifying the patient that a choice exists), Option Talk (discussing alternatives), and Decision Talk (supporting the patient to explore preferences and reach a decision). This approach honours the ethical principle of autonomy and ensures that the clinical path aligns with the patient's lived reality.

The Three Pillars of the Alliance

According to the Bordin (1979) model, which is highly applicable to medicine, the therapeutic alliance consists of three essential components:

Agreement on Goals: What are we trying to achieve? (e.g., curing the disease vs. maintaining quality of life).

Agreement on Tasks: What are the steps to get there? (e.g., adherence to medication, lifestyle changes).

The Bond: The underlying trust and interpersonal connection that sustains the relationship during difficult times.

Case Study 4.1: The Hesitant Oncology Patient

Mr. J, a 68-year-old retired teacher, was diagnosed with Stage III lung cancer. The standard of care was aggressive chemotherapy. However, Mr. J was hesitant, haunted by memories of his wife's difficult journey with the same treatment years prior. Instead of pushing the protocol, his oncologist, Dr. S, employed active listening. 'Tell me what worries you most,' Dr. S asked. Mr. J expressed that he valued being lucid and alert for his grandson's upcoming graduation more than a slight statistical increase in survival. By discussing palliative care and adjuvant options without judgment, they reached a consensus on a lower-intensity regimen. This plan honoured both clinical goals and personal quality of life, leading to high treatment adherence and a peaceful final chapter for the patient.

Navigating Barriers to Rapport

Building a therapeutic alliance is not always seamless. Several factors can impede the connection:

Time Constraints: The 'efficiency paradox' often leads clinicians to interrupt patients within the first 18 seconds of speaking. Research suggests that if allowed to speak for just 60 seconds without interruption, most patients will disclose their primary concern, ultimately saving time (Beckman & Frankel, 1984).

Technology: The 'electronic health record (EHR) barrier'—where the clinician stares at the screen instead of the patient—distracts from the human bond. Practitioners must master 'eye-contact-to-screen' ratios.

Clinical Arrogance: The belief that medical knowledge supersedes the patient's subjective experience of their own body.

Cultural Competence and Global Health Perspectives

In a globalized world, clinical excellence requires cultural humility. Trust is often filtered through the lens of a patient's cultural background, historical experiences with the medical system, and spiritual beliefs. For example, in many African and Southern African contexts, the concept of 'Ubuntu'—I am because we are—means that healthcare decisions are often communal rather than individual. A clinician who ignores the family's role in a patient's care may inadvertently fracture the therapeutic alliance (Mabuza, 2022). Building trust with marginalized populations requires acknowledging past systemic biases and demonstrating a commitment to equity. Rapport is built when the patient feels that the doctor is an ally against the disease, not a representative of a cold bureaucracy.

"People don't care how much you know until they know how much you care."

— *Theodore Roosevelt*

The Role of Non-Verbal Communication

Communication is 7% verbal, 38% vocal, and 55% non-verbal. The 'SOLER' acronym serves as a helpful guide for maintaining rapport: - S: Sit squarely (conveying interest). - O: Open posture (non-defensive). -

L: Lean toward the patient. - E: Eye contact (culturally appropriate). - R: Relax (conveying confidence and calm).

Repairing a Fractured Alliance

Rapport is not static; it can be broken by misunderstandings, medical errors, or perceived slights. Clinical mastery involves the ability to recognize these 'ruptures' and initiate repair. Acknowledging a patient's frustration, apologizing for a delay, or simply saying, 'I sense that we are not on the same page; let's restart,' can often strengthen the alliance more than if the rupture had never occurred (Safran & Muran, 2000).

The Impact of Continuity of Care

Trust is a longitudinal asset. While a single encounter can establish rapport, a deep therapeutic alliance is forged over time. Patients with a long-term relationship with a primary provider report higher levels of trust and are significantly more likely to follow through with screenings and preventative care. In the era of fragmented specialized medicine, the physician must act as the steward of the patient's narrative, ensuring that the person is not lost in a sea of data points.

Case Study 4.2: The 'Difficult' Patient

Ms. L was labelled 'difficult' and 'non-compliant' by several departments for refusing to take her hypertension medication. Upon referral, Dr. Mabuza chose not to lecture her. Instead, he spent the first 15 minutes of the visit talking about her life in rural Eswatini. He discovered she believed the medication caused bad dreams that were spiritually significant. By acknowledging the validity of her spiritual concerns and switching to a different class of medication with a late-night dosing schedule, the 'difficult' patient became fully compliant. The breakthrough was not pharmacological; it was relational.

Summary and Conclusion

The therapeutic alliance is the foundation upon which all clinical excellence is built. It requires a blend of emotional intelligence, cultural humility, and ethical commitment. By mastering the art of the alliance, the clinician does more than treat symptoms; they honour the dignity of the human person and fulfil the true calling of the medical profession.

References

Balint, M. (1957). The Doctor, His Patient and the Illness. Pitman Medical Publishing.

Beckman, H. B., & Frankel, R. M. (1984). The effect of physician behavior on the collection of data. Annals of Internal Medicine.

Bordin, E. S. (1979). The generalizability of the psychoanalytic concept of the working alliance. Psychotherapy: Theory, Research & Practice.

Charles, C., Gafni, A., & Whelan, T. (1997). Shared decision-making in the medical encounter: what does it mean? Social Science & Medicine.

Decety, J., & Fotopoulou, A. (2015). Why empathy has a beneficial impact on others in medicine. Frontiers in Behavioral Neuroscience.

Halpern, J. (2003). What is Clinical Empathy? Journal of General Internal Medicine.

Mabuza, M. (2022). Medicine and Sociology of Health.

Safran, J. D., & Muran, J. C. (2000). Negotiating the Therapeutic Alliance: A Relational Treatment Guide.

Chapter 5: Navigating Ethical Dilemmas: Principles and Case Studies in Medical Ethics

LEARNING OBJECTIVES

After studying this chapter, you should be able to:

- Define and apply the four foundational pillars of biomedical ethics.
- Utilize the "Four-Box Method" for structured ethical case analysis.
- Identify emerging ethical challenges in AI and genomic medicine (CRISPR).
- Distinguish between legal requirements and moral obligations in clinical practice.
- Recognize the signs of moral distress and the importance of ethical resilience.

Medical ethics is not a static set of rules but a living, breathing framework that evolves alongside humanity. In the quiet corridors of a hospital, ethics is the silent witness to every decision made. As we advance into an era of genomic medicine and artificial intelligence, the complexity of these decisions scales exponentially.

Dr. Pellegrino once noted that medicine is the 'most humane of sciences and the most scientific of humanities' (Pellegrino, 1979). To achieve clinical mastery, a physician must be as skilled in moral reasoning as they are in surgical technique.

The Four Pillars: A Moral Compass

The foundational pillars of biomedical ethics serve as the primary compass for resolving conflicts in care (Beauchamp & Childress, 2019):

Autonomy: This principle recognizes the patient's right to self-determination. In modern practice, this has shifted the physician's role from a paternalistic authority to a partner in care. It requires that patients are given truthful information to make informed choices.

Beneficence: The duty to act in the best interest of the patient. This goes beyond 'not hurting' and requires proactive steps to contribute to the patient's welfare.

Non-maleficence: Primum non nocere (First, do no harm). This principle demands that the risks of a treatment must not outweigh the benefits, particularly in experimental or highly invasive procedures.

Justice: Often the most overlooked, justice involves the fair distribution of benefits, risks, and costs. In a world of finite resources, justice asks: 'Is this treatment accessible to all, and is its use for one patient depriving another of a life-saving intervention?'

The Four-Box Method and Emerging Dilemmas

Ethics is not merely about feelings; it is a rigorous discipline. Using the 'four-box' method allows for a structured approach to cases where emotions often run high (Jonsen, Siegler, & Winslade, 2015):

Medical Indications: What are the goals of treatment? What is the probability of success? (Principles of Beneficence and Non-maleficence).

Patient Preferences: Has the patient expressed prior wishes? Is their consent informed and voluntary? (Principle of Autonomy).

Quality of Life: What is the prospect, with or without treatment, for a return to the patient's normal life? (Principles of Beneficence, Non-maleficence, and Autonomy).

Contextual Features: Are there family issues, provider conflicts, or financial factors? (Principle of Justice).

The Practitioner's Note: In medical ethics, the 'correct' path is rarely the easiest one. We must differentiate between legal requirements and moral obligations.

Ethics in the Age of Technology

We are currently navigating a 'Digital Frontier' in medicine. The use of AI in diagnostics raises questions of 'Algorithmic Justice.' If a machine makes a mistake based on biased data, who is responsible? Furthermore, the rise of CRISPR technology forces us to ask if we are treating disease or redesigning the human condition.

Case Study 1: The 'Gentle Death' Dilemma

A 78-year-old grandfather, Mr. Thompson, suffered multi-organ failure. His family requested maximum life-sustaining treatment. However, the medical team concluded these were 'non-beneficial'—only prolonging the dying process. Reflection: The conflict lies between the family's autonomy and the physician's duty of non-maleficence. By transitioning to palliative care, the team honoured the patient's dignity.

Practitioner's Reflection: Ethical Resilience

Clinical excellence requires 'moral courage.' It is easy to follow a protocol; it is difficult to challenge a senior colleague when you believe a patient's autonomy is being compromised. Ethical mastery also involves recognizing 'Moral Distress,' which occurs when a physician knows the right thing to do but is prevented by institutional constraints.

"The good physician treats the disease; the great physician treats the patient who has the disease." — Sir William Osler

"In the face of suffering, the best medicine is sometimes not a drug, but the presence of another human being who honours your story." — Dr. Mbuso Mabuza

References:

Beauchamp, T. L., & Childress, J. F. (2019). Principles of Biomedical Ethics (8th ed.). Oxford University Press.

Jonsen, A. R., Siegler, M., & Winslade, W. J. (2015). Clinical Ethics: A Practical Approach to Ethical Decisions in Clinical Medicine (8th ed.). McGraw-Hill Education.

Osler, W. (n.d.). Quotations in Medicine.

Pellegrino, E. D. (1979). Humanism and the Physician. University of Tennessee Press.

Chapter 6: Communication Skills: The Cornerstone of Effective Patient Care

"The single biggest problem in communication is the illusion that it has taken place." — George Bernard Shaw

Learning Objectives

By the end of this chapter, readers will be able to:

- Define the role of 'narrative competence' in modern clinical practice.
- Identify and translate medical jargon into 'living room language' for better patient understanding.
- Apply the SPIKES protocol to deliver life-altering diagnoses with compassion.
- Utilize the NURSE mnemonic to address and validate patient emotions.
- Implement 'The Golden Minute' and 'Teach-Back' methods to improve diagnostic accuracy and patient adherence.
- Explain the ethical relationship between effective communication and the principle of patient autonomy.

In the high-stakes arena of modern medicine, where robotic surgery and genomic sequencing often dominate the headlines, it is easy to overlook the most fundamental tool in a physician's armamentarium: the spoken word. Effective communication is not a 'soft skill' to be applied when time permits; it is a clinical skill as essential as physical examination or surgical technique. It is the bridge between a diagnosis and a cure, the medium through which trust is built, and the primary safeguard against diagnostic error.

Research consistently demonstrates that superior communication correlates with better clinical outcomes, including improved physiological markers such as blood pressure and glucose control, as well as higher rates of patient adherence to treatment plans. Conversely, poor communication is the leading root cause of sentinel events and malpractice litigation. To achieve clinical mastery, the practitioner must move beyond the transactional exchange of data and embrace the relational art of human connection.

1. The Foundations of Dialogue

The medical interview serves two purposes: gathering information to reach an accurate diagnosis and establishing a therapeutic relationship. Mastery in the former is useless without success in the latter.

The Power of Narrative Medicine: Rita Charon (2001) pioneered the concept of Narrative Medicine, arguing that clinicians need 'narrative competence'—the ability to acknowledge, absorb, interpret, and be moved by the stories of illness. Instead of rushing to a checklist of symptoms, the clinician should start with open-ended inquiries: "Tell me about what has been happening." This allows the patient to frame their experience, revealing psychological stressors or social determinants that a rigid 'Review of Systems' would ignore.

Avoiding the Jargon Trap: Medical jargon acts as a barrier, not a bridge. Terms like 'idiopathic,' 'ambulatory,' or 'negative results' often carry different meanings for patients. Masterful communicators translate complex pathophysiology into 'living room language.'

2. Breaking Bad News: The SPIKES Protocol

Delivering a life-altering diagnosis is perhaps the most daunting task a physician faces. The SPIKES protocol (Baile et al., 2000) provides a structured, compassionate framework:

S – Setting up the Interview: Privacy is non-negotiable. Arrange the room so there are no physical barriers. Sit down to signal that you are not in a rush.

P – Assessing Perception: Before giving information, find out what the patient already knows. "What is your understanding of why we did these scans?"

I – Obtaining Invitation: Asking "Would you like me to go over the details of the results now?" gives the patient a sense of control.

K – Giving Knowledge: Avoid 'the blunt force trauma' of direct bad news. Use 'warning shots' like, "I'm afraid I have some difficult news to share."

E – Addressing Emotions with Empathy: Use the NURSE mnemonic: Name the emotion, Understand it, Respect the patient, Support them, and Explore the feeling further.

S – Strategy and Summary: Outline a clear plan: "Here are our next steps. We will see the oncologist on Tuesday."

Case Study: The Young Father and the Weight of Truth

Dr. Mbuso Mabuza was tasked with informing 'David,' a 34-year-old father of two, that his persistent back pain was metastatic Stage IV lung cancer. Utilizing the SPIKES protocol, Dr. Mabuza ensured the setting was quiet. When assessing David's perception, he realized David thought he just had a slipped disc. After the 'warning shot,' Dr. Mabuza delivered the news gently. David went silent for several minutes. Instead of filling the silence with medical statistics, Dr. Mabuza waited, finally saying, "I can see how overwhelming this is." This empathetic witness allowed David to eventually ask, "How do I tell my wife?" By the end of the hour, David left with a plan and the knowledge that his doctor was walking beside him.

3. The Art of Deep Listening

Active listening involves the 'Golden Minute.' Studies show that if a doctor allows a patient to speak uninterrupted for just sixty seconds at the start of an encounter, the patient will usually disclose the primary reason for their visit (Beckman & Frankel, 1984).

The Teach-Back Method: To ensure the patient is an equal partner, use the 'teach-back' method. Instead of asking "Do you understand?", ask "To make sure I've explained this clearly, how would you describe the plan to your spouse when you get home?"

Reflections on Ethical Presence

Clinical mastery requires us to be present not just as technicians, but as human beings. The ethical core of communication lies in the principle of Autonomy. We cannot respect a patient's autonomy if we have not facilitated their understanding. Communication is the vehicle for Informed Consent—it is not a signature on a form, but a shared journey toward a decision that aligns with the patient's values.

"To cure sometimes, to relieve often, to comfort always." — 15th Century Proverb

References

Baile, W. F., et al. (2000). SPIKES—A Six Step Protocol for Delivering Bad News. The Oncologist.

Beckman, H. B., & Frankel, R. M. (1984). The Effect of Physician Behavior on the Collection of Data. Annals of Internal Medicine.

Charon, R. (2001). Narrative Medicine: A Model for Empathy, Reflection, Profession, and Trust. JAMA.

Epstein, R. M., & Gramling, R. E. (2013). What is Shared Decision Making? Patient Education and Counseling.

Stewart, M., et al. (2003). Patient-Centered Medicine: Transforming the Clinical Method. Radcliffe Medical Press.

Chapter 7: Cultural Competence: Providing Equitable Care to Diverse Populations

Learning Objectives

- Define cultural competence, cultural humility, and clinical equity within a modern healthcare framework.
- Identify and mitigate the impact of implicit bias on diagnostic accuracy and patient outcomes.
- Master the application of the LEARN model in complex cross-cultural patient encounters.
- Evaluate the role of social determinants of health and linguistic barriers in creating health disparities.
- Formulate strategies for integrating traditional beliefs with evidence-based medical practice.

In the modern clinical landscape, the stethoscope and the scalpel are often secondary to the most powerful tool in a physician's arsenal: the ability to understand. As medicine becomes increasingly globalized, the 'standard' patient no longer exists. Cultural competence is not merely a 'soft skill' or a checkbox for hospital accreditation; it is a clinical exigency. It is the bridge between a correct diagnosis and a successful therapeutic outcome.

Betancourt et al. (2003) argue that cultural competence is a necessary strategy to eliminate racial and ethnic disparities in health care. This chapter explores how to move beyond static 'cultural facts' toward a dynamic, reflexive practice that honours the humanity of every individual who enters the consultation room.

The Invisible Barrier: Implicit Bias and Self Awareness

Even the most dedicated clinicians harbour unconscious biases—automatic associations that influence our perceptions and actions without our permission. FitzGerald and Hurst (2017) demonstrated that implicit bias significantly affects clinical judgment, frequently leading to under-prescribing of pain medication for minority populations or lower rates of referral for specialized procedures.

Reflexive practice is the antidote. It requires the clinician to pause and ask: 'What assumptions am I making about this patient based on their appearance, accent, or background?' As Dr. Vivianne Idriss once said, 'We do not see the world as it is; we see it as we are.' Recognizing our own 'cultural lens' is the first step toward clinical excellence.

"Cultural humility is not a destination; it is a way of being—a lifelong commitment to self-evaluation and self-critique." — Unknown

Actionable Frameworks: The LEARN Model

To move from theory to practice, clinicians need a scaffolding for communication. The LEARN Model (Berlin and Fowkes, 1983) provides a robust framework:

- Listen with empathy and understanding to the patient's perception of the problem.
- Explain your perceptions of the problem and the strategy for treatment.
- Acknowledge and discuss the differences and similarities between these perceptions.
- Recommend treatment while involving the patient in the process.
- Negotiate agreement.

Case Study: Bridging Two Worlds in Diabetes Management

Thabo, a 55-year-old man from a rural community, was consistently non-adherent to his insulin regimen. Upon using the LEARN model, his physician discovered that Thabo believed his illness was a 'spiritual calling' that required cleansing by a traditional healer (Sangoma). Instead of dismissing the belief, the physician invited the healer to a consultation. They agreed that the 'cleansing herbs' would be taken in the morning, and the insulin in the evening. By respecting the healer's role, the physician gained Thabo's trust. Within six months, his blood sugar was stabilized. This synergy—rather than conflict—saved Thabo's life.

Linguistic Competence and the Power of Voice

Language is the vehicle of care. Research indicates that patients with limited English proficiency (LEP) are more likely to experience adverse medical events (Flores, 2005). Relying on family members—especially children—to interpret is not only unethical but clinically dangerous. Professional medical interpreters provide not just word-for-word translation, but cultural brokering that can illuminate a patient's hidden fears.

Structural Competency: Beyond the Individual

Structural competency asks us to look at the forces that shape health before the patient even reaches the clinic. Neighbourhood safety, food security, and historical injustices play a profound role (Metzl & Hansen, 2014). An excellent clinician understands that a patient's 'non-compliance' might be an 'inability to access' due to structural barriers.

Reflective Exercise:

Reflection: Think of a time you felt misunderstood by a person in authority. How did that affect your willingness to cooperate? Now, apply that feeling to a patient who feels alienated by the clinical environment.

References

Berlin, E. A., & Fowkes, W. C. (1983). A teaching framework for cross-cultural health care. Western Journal of Medicine.

Betancourt, J. R., et al. (2003). Cultural competence in health care. Field Report, Commonwealth Fund.

FitzGerald, C., & Hurst, S. (2017). Implicit bias in healthcare professionals: a systematic review. BMC Medical Ethics.

Flores, G. (2005). The impact of medical interpreter services on the quality of health care. Medical Care Research and Review.

Metzl, J. M., & Hansen, H. (2014). Structural competency: Theorizing a new medical engagement. Social Science & Medicine.

Chapter 8: Quality Improvement: Measuring and Enhancing Patient Outcomes

LEARNING OBJECTIVES

- Define Quality Improvement (QI) within the context of clinical excellence.
- Apply the Donabedian Model (Structure, Process, Outcome) to clinical settings.
- Synthesize the Plan-Do-Study-Act (PDSA) cycle for localized problem-solving.
- Evaluate the role of multidisciplinary teams in driving sustainable healthcare changes.
- Internalize the ethical imperative of continuous improvement in patient safety.

In the pursuit of clinical mastery, one must recognize that excellence is not a static destination but a dynamic trajectory. Quality Improvement (QI) represents the systematic and continuous actions that lead to measurable improvement in healthcare services. For the clinician, QI is the bridge between theoretical knowledge and the actual health status of the community. As we navigate the complexities of modern medicine, the ability to critique our own systems becomes as vital as the ability to diagnose a rare disease.

Clinicians often view Quality Improvement (QI) as a bureaucratic necessity—a series of forms to be filled or boxes to be checked. However, within the framework of Clinical Mastery, QI is the heartbeat of professional accountability. It is the realization that being a 'good doctor' is insufficient if the system in which you operate prevents your patients from achieving optimal recovery.

The Theoretical Foundation: Structure, Process, and Outcome

The cornerstone of modern QI is the Donabedian Model (Donabedian, 1988). Donabedian proposed that quality can be evaluated through three lenses: Structure (the environment and resources), Process (the actions taken), and Outcomes (the end result for the patient). While clinical mastery often focuses on 'Process'—how we treat—true excellence requires us to link these processes relentlessly to 'Outcomes'. If our mortality rates do not drop or patient satisfaction does not rise, our refined processes are merely academic exercises.

Donabedian's framework (1988) reminds us that excellent outcomes are not accidental. If we look at surgical mortality, for instance, we must evaluate the Structure (Is the theatre equipped with modern pulse oximeters?), the Process (Does the surgical team follow the WHO Safe Surgery Checklist?), and finally, the Outcome (What is the 30-day post-operative mortality rate?). A master clinician understands that improvements in the structure and process are the only reliable levers for shifting the outcome.

"Quality is never an accident; it is always the result of high intention, sincere effort, intelligent direction and skilful execution. — William A. Foster"

The Engine of Change: The PDSA Cycle

The Plan-Do-Study-Act (PDSA) cycle is the scientific method applied to management. 'Plan' involves identifying a goal and a theory of change. 'Do' is the implementation on a small, manageable scale. 'Study' involves the rigorous analysis of data collected during the test. Finally, 'Act' involves refining the change based on what was learned (Moen & Norman, 2010).

CASE STUDY: The Surgical Infection Breakthrough

In a prominent regional hospital, a surgical team noted a stagnant post-operative infection rate. By applying Lean methodologies—a system derived from manufacturing that focuses on eliminating waste—the team discovered that preoperative antibiotics were often administered too late to be effective. Through three PDSA cycles, they redesigned the workflow, placing the responsibility on the anaesthesia team to trigger the dose exactly 60 minutes before the first incision. The result: a 30% reduction in infections over six months.

Lean and Six Sigma in the Clinical Setting

Beyond PDSA, Lean and Six Sigma provide advanced frameworks. Six Sigma focuses on reducing variability. In medicine, variability is the enemy of safety. Lean, conversely, removes 'Muda' (waste), such as unnecessary waiting times for diagnostic imaging, which directly impacts patient anxiety and outcomes. In the Lean philosophy, waste is anything that does not add value to the patient's journey.

"Every system is perfectly designed to get the results it gets. — Paul Batalden"

Patient-Cantered Outcomes: The True North

Quality is not solely defined by the clinician. Patient-Reported Outcome Measures (PROMs) and Patient-Reported Experience Measures (PREMs) are essential. Excellence means asking: 'Did the surgery allow you to return to the activities you love?' rather than just 'Is the wound healed?' (Porter et al., 2016).

Reflective Exercise

Reflective Practice: Consider your last clinical shift. Was there a bottleneck that frustrated you? That frustration is the seeds of a QI project. Actionable Insight: Identify one recurring delay in your clinic this week. What is one 'small-scale' change you could test using a PDSA methodology to address it?

References and Further Reading

Donabedian, A. (1988). The quality of care: How can it be assessed? JAMA, 260(12), 1743-1748.

Moen, R. D., & Norman, C. L. (2010). Evolution of the PDSA cycle. Quality Progress, 43(11), 22.

Porter, M. E., Larsson, S., & Lee, T. H. (2016). Standardizing patient outcomes measurement. New England Journal of Medicine, 374(6), 504-506.

Pronovost, P., et al. (2006). An intervention to decrease catheter-related bloodstream infections in the ICU. NEJM, 355(26), 2725-2732.

Chapter 9: Patient Safety: Minimizing Errors and Adverse Events

LEARNING OBJECTIVES

After completing this chapter, readers should be able to:

- Analyse the systemic nature of medical errors using the Swiss Cheese Model.
- Differentiate between human error, at-risk behaviour, and reckless behaviour within a Just Culture framework.
- Implement practical safety tools such as surgical time-outs and structured communication (SBAR).
- Foster a non-hierarchical environment where patient safety is a shared responsibility.

"The first rule of medicine is 'Primum non nocere'—First, do no harm."
— HIPPOCRATIC OATH

Patient safety is not merely a technical requirement; it is the moral bedrock of clinical excellence. In the high-stakes environment of modern medicine, the prevention of errors and adverse effects is a continuous, dynamic process. As we transition from an era of "blame and shame" to one of systemic resilience, we recognize that excellence in medicine is defined as much by what we prevent as by what we treat.

The Swiss Cheese Model: Understanding System Failure

James Reason's 'Swiss Cheese Model' remains the gold standard for understanding how complex systems fail. In this model, an organization's defences against failure are likened to a series of slices of Swiss cheese, stacked side by side (Reason, 2000).

The Anatomy of a System Failure:

The Slices: Represent layers of defence (e.g., protocols, technology, clinical checklists, experienced staff).

The Holes: Represent "active failures" (unsafe acts by frontline personnel) and "latent conditions" (systemic weaknesses like understaffing or poor equipment design).

Alignment: When the holes in many layers momentarily align, a "trajectory of accident opportunity" is created, allowing a hazard to pass through all defences and reach the patient.

This model shifts the focus from the individual at the "sharp end" of care to the system as a whole. It suggests that instead of trying to change human nature (which is prone to error), we must change the conditions under which humans work.

Clinical Reflection: Think of a near-miss you witnessed recently. What were the "holes" in the system that allowed it to get as far as it did? More importantly, what was the "slice of cheese" that finally stopped it?

Just Culture: Moving Beyond Blame

A 'Just Culture' is the middle ground between a culture of blame and a culture of total immunity. Today, we recognize that to improve safety, we must encourage the reporting of near-misses and errors without fear of unjust retribution (Kohn et al., 2000).

Case Study: The Empowerment of a Junior Nurse

In a busy metropolitan hospital, a surgical team was preparing for a knee replacement. A junior nurse noticed that the consent form indicated the right leg while the registrar pointed to the left. Because the department had fostered a Just Culture, she felt empowered to "stop the line." A catastrophic "wrong-site" surgery was avoided. The surgeon later publicly thanked the nurse, reinforcing that safety is everyone's job.

The Three Behaviours in Just Culture:

1. Human Error: Inadvertent slips or lapses. Management: Console the individual and fix the system.

2. At-Risk Behaviour: Shortcuts taken to be "efficient." Management: Coach the individual to see the hidden risks.

3. Reckless Behaviour: Conscious disregard of risk. Management: Discipline the individual.

Practical Strategies for Clinical Mastery

1. Structured Communication (SBAR): The Situation, Background, Assessment, Recommendation framework ensures that critical information is conveyed concisely.

2. The WHO Surgical Safety Checklist: This checklist has been shown to reduce surgical complications by up to 36% and mortality by 47% (Haynes et al., 2009).

Conclusion: The Path Forward

Excellence in medicine is a journey, not a destination. By embracing the principles of patient safety—acknowledging our fallibility, building resilient systems, and fostering a culture where every voice is heard—we honour our commitment to our patients.

"Safety is not the absence of accidents; it is the presence of capacity."
— TODD CONKLIN, PHD

References

Haynes, A. B., et al. (2009). A surgical safety checklist to reduce morbidity and mortality in a global population. New England Journal of Medicine.

Kohn, L. T., et al. (2000). To Err Is Human: Building a Safer Health System. National Academies Press.

Reason, J. (2000). Human error: models and management. BMJ.

World Health Organization (2023). Patient Safety: Global Action on Patient Safety. WHO Fact Sheets.

Chapter 10: Leadership in Medicine: Inspiring and Empowering Healthcare Teams

Learning Objectives

- Define the concept of distributed leadership within the clinical context.
- Articulate the role of Emotional Intelligence (EQ) in conflict resolution and team cohesion.
- Identify strategies for fostering psychological safety in high-stakes medical environments.
- Analyse the impact of leadership styles on patient safety and clinical outcomes.

Every physician is a leader. Leadership in medicine is not merely an administrative title but a clinical competency—the ability to influence others to work toward a common goal: the best possible patient care. In the modern healthcare landscape, technical brilliance alone is insufficient. Mastery requires the ability to navigate the complex human systems that deliver that technical care.

The Philosophy of Physician Leadership

The traditional medical hierarchy is evolving. Historically, the 'captain of the ship' model placed the physician at the apex, issuing commands. While clear lines of authority remain vital in crisis (e.g., a cardiac arrest), the broader movement of modern healthcare favours a 'collaborative mastery' approach. As Dr. Mbuso Mabuza posits, 'Clinical excellence is a team sport; the physician's role is to coach, inspire, and synchronize the players.'

Emotional Intelligence (EQ): The Hidden Competency

High clinical IQ is not enough for medical excellence. Research by Daniel Goleman (1995) popularized the concept that Emotional Intelligence (EQ)—consisting of self-awareness, self-regulation, motivation, empathy, and social skill—is a more accurate predictor of leadership success than technical skill.

Edmondson (1999) introduced 'Psychological Safety'—a belief that one will not be punished for speaking up with ideas, questions, or mistakes. This is the cornerstone of high-performing healthcare teams.

"Leadership is not about being in charge. It is about taking care of those in your charge."

— Simon Sinek

Distributed Leadership: Power in Partnership

Effective leadership in medicine is often distributed, where different team members take the lead based on their expertise rather than their formal rank. This model reduces the cognitive load on the physician and empowers the entire team to take ownership of patient outcomes.

Case Study: The Transformation of Unit 4B

Dr. Thompson assumed leadership of an Emergency Department (ED) plagued by high staff turnover and frequent near misses. Key Interventions included 'After-Action Reviews' focusing on systems, open-door hours, and transparent decision-making. Outcome: Within 18 months, staff retention increased by 40% as Dr. Thompson moved from being 'The Boss' to 'The Facilitator'.

Communication and the Anatomy of Conflict

The currency of leadership is communication. West et al. (2014) demonstrated that well-functioning teams have lower patient mortality rates. A clinical leader uses interest-based negotiation: focusing on the common interest (the patient) rather than the 'position' (the ego).

Reflective Practice: Think of a time you witnessed a breakdown in team communication. How did the hierarchy impact the outcome? What could a leadership intervention have changed?

Mentorship and Legacy

True medical leaders create more leaders, not more followers. Mentorship is the intentional development of the next generation of physicians. In conclusion, professional excellence in medicine is inseparable from leadership. To lead is to serve.

References

Edmondson, A. (1999). Psychological Safety and Learning Behavior in Work Teams. Administrative Science Quarterly.

Fitzgerald, L., et al. (2013). Distributed leadership in healthcare: The barriers and facilitators. Journal of Health Organization and Management.

Goleman, D. (1995). Emotional Intelligence: Why It Can Matter More Than IQ. Bantam Books.

West, M. A., et al. (2014). The link between management and clinical outcomes in the NHS. The Lancet.

Chapter 11: Technology and Innovation: Harnessing Advances for Better Patient Care

Learning Objectives

- Evaluate the impact of Artificial Intelligence (AI) and Machine Learning (ML) on clinical decision support.
- Analyse the role of Electronic Health Records (EHR) and wearable technology in proactive patient management.
- Assess the ethics of data privacy and the 'digital divide' in modern medicine.
- Develop strategies for maintaining the 'human touch' in a technologically mediated clinical environment.
- Understand the logistical and clinical benefits of telemedicine and remote patient monitoring (RPM).

In the modern era, the stethoscope is no longer the sole symbol of medical practice. It has been joined, and sometimes surpassed, by algorithms, sensors, and high-definition screens. Eric Topol (2019) argues in 'Deep Medicine' that the greatest potential of technology is not to replace the physician but to provide the gift of time—allowing doctors to be more human. However, mastery in this digital landscape requires a delicate balance between technical proficiency and empathetic presence.

The Digital Health Revolution: Data as a Diagnostic Tool

The transition from paper charts to Electronic Health Records (EHRs) was the first tremor of a massive shift. Today, we move beyond static data to dynamic data streams. Wearable technology—from smartwatches that detect atrial fibrillation to continuous glucose monitors (CGM)—provides a longitudinal view of patient health that a single clinic visit never could.

"The computer should not be a barrier between the doctor and the patient, but a window into the patient's biological reality."

The primary challenge is information overload. Clinicians today are often 'data-rich but insight-poor.' Data privacy, governed by frameworks like HIPAA and GDPR, is no longer just a legal requirement but a fundamental part of the patient-provider trust (Mittelstadt, 2017).

Artificial Intelligence: The New Clinical Partner

Artificial Intelligence is redefining diagnostics, particularly in image-heavy fields like radiology, dermatology, and pathology. Predictive analytics is increasingly used to identify patients at risk of sepsis before clinical deterioration becomes manifest. This proactive stance represents a fundamental shift in the physician's role—becoming a pilot who navigates using both visual cues and radar.

Breaking Barriers: Telemedicine

Telemedicine has evolved from a pandemic-necessity to a permanent pillar of accessibility. Accessibility is not merely about physical distance; it is about social inclusion. For the elderly or single parents, the video check-in is a bridge to health equity.

Case Study: The Rural Heart Failure Initiative

In a remote district in Eswatini, a clinic integrated cellular-connected scales and pulse oximeters for 100 high-risk heart failure patients. By intervening with oral diuretic adjustments via phone when alerts were triggered, the clinic reduced hospital readmissions by 40% over 12 months. This success story underscores how innovation can solve complex delivery problems in resource-limited settings.

Preserving the Human Element in a Digital World

As we embrace innovation, the risk of 'technological dehumanization' grows. A doctor staring at an EHR screen throughout a consultation may miss the subtle tear in a patient's eye.

Reflection for the Practitioner

Reflection: How many times during your last shift did a digital tool improve your connection with a patient? How many times did it hinder it? Think about a patient who felt 'unheard' despite you having all their data on your screen.

Ethical Considerations and Innovation

Algorithmic Bias: Ensuring AI models are trained on diverse populations.

The Digital Divide: Preventing a tiered healthcare system.

Right to Explanation: Patients deserve to know when an algorithm is influencing their care.

"Innovation distinguishes between a leader and a follower." — Steve Jobs

Concluding Thoughts: The Augmented Physician

The mastery of clinical practice in the 21st century is defined by the synergy of machine intelligence and human intuition. We must avoid 'technological determinism' and always return to the bedside where the true essence of healing resides.

References and Further Reading

Mittelstadt, B. (2017). Ethics of Health Care Robotics. Theoretical Medicine and Bioethics.

Topol, E. (2019). Deep Medicine: How Artificial Intelligence Can Make Healthcare Human Again.

Wosik, J., et al. (2020). Telehealth transformation: COVID-19 and the rise of virtual care.

Zuboff, S. (2019). The Age of Surveillance Capitalism.

Chapter 12: Preventing Burnout and Promoting Well-being in Medical Practice

"The expectation that we can be immersed in suffering and loss daily and not be touched by it is as unrealistic as expecting to be able to walk through water without getting wet." — Rachel Naomi Remen

In the high-stakes world of medicine, the focus is almost exclusively on the patient. However, the integrity of the healthcare system rests upon the shoulders of its clinicians. Physician burnout is not just a personal struggle; it is a systemic epidemic that threatens the very foundation of clinical excellence. To practice 'Excellence in Medicine,' one must recognize that the longevity of a medical career is predicated on the clinician's own mental, emotional, and physical well-being.

LEARNING OBJECTIVES

- Identify the three cardinal dimensions of burnout as defined by the Maslach Burnout Inventory (MBI).
- Analyse the systemic and individual factors contributing to moral injury and compassion fatigue.
- Develop a personalized 'Resilience Toolkit' incorporating evidence-based mindfulness and boundary-setting strategies.
- Understand the ethical imperative of self-care as a component of professional duty to patients.
- Implement peer-support frameworks within a clinical department to foster a culture of well-being.

Recognizing the Signs: The Anatomy of Burnout

Burnout in medicine is often misunderstood as simple "stress" or "exhaustion." Research by Maslach et al. (2001) defines it as a profound occupational syndrome. It manifests through three distinct pillars:

Emotional Exhaustion: A feeling of being overextended and depleted of one's emotional and physical resources.

Depersonalization (Cynicism): Treating patients as objects or diagnoses. This leads to a significant decline in quality of care.

Low Personal Accomplishment: A tendency to evaluate oneself negatively and feel ineffective.

Reflective Exercise: Take a moment to scan your last week. Did you find yourself retreating into cynicism to survive a shift? Recognizing this is not a sign of weakness, but a biological signal that your empathy reserves are depleted.

Systemic Drivers and Moral Injury

Talbot and Dean (2018) introduced the concept of 'Moral Injury' in medicine. Unlike burnout, which suggests a failure of the individual to cope, moral injury occurs when clinicians are repeatedly forced to make choices that transgress their deeply held commitment to healing—such as prioritizing billing over bedside time.

Real-Life Example: The Administrative Trap

Consider Dr. A, an oncologist who spends 4 hours on electronic health records (EHR) for every 1 hour spent with patients. Administrative burden is a leading predictor of physician attrition (West et al., 2018).

Self-Care as a Professional Duty

Resilience Tactics:

- Mindfulness-Based Stress Reduction (MBSR): 10 minutes can reduce cortisol levels.
- Boundaries and the 'Power of No': Setting limits is essential for long-term mastery.
- The Buddy System: Transitioning from a 'lone wolf' mentality to a 'communal' one.

Extended Case Study: The Resident Buddy System

Dr. L implemented a 'Buddy System' where residents performed 48-hour 'pulse checks.' If a buddy signalled 'amber' or 'red,' others covered tasks to allow a 15-minute break. This intervention reduced reports of severe exhaustion by 30% over six months.

Conclusion and Future Directions

Excellence in medicine is a marathon, not a sprint. To reach the pinnacle of clinical mastery, you must preserve the instrument of your craft: yourself.

References

Krasner, M. S., et al. (2009). Association of mindful communication with burnout. JAMA.

Maslach, C., et al. (2001). Job burnout. Annual Review of Psychology.

Shanafelt, T. D., et al. (2012). Burnout and satisfaction with work-life balance. Archives of Internal Medicine.

Talbot, S. G., & Dean, W. (2018). Physicians are not burning out. They are suffering from moral injury. STAT News.

West, C. P., et al. (2018). Interventions to prevent and reduce physician burnout: a systematic review. The Lancet.

Chapter 13: The Doctor as a Lifelong Learner: Continuous Professional Development

Learning Objectives:

After studying this chapter, the reader will be able to:

- Analyse the shifting paradigm of medical knowledge and the necessity of lifelong learning in the 21st century.
- Implement effective self-directed learning (SDL) strategies based on real-world clinical encounters.
- Develop advanced skills in the critical appraisal of biomedical literature using Evidence-Based Medicine (EBM) frameworks.
- Reflect on the intersection of professional development, doctor well-being, and patient safety.
- Cultivate a mindset of 'Curiosity-Driven Practice' to prevent cognitive stagnation and burnout.

Medical knowledge is estimated to double every few months. In this environment, the medical degree is not the end of education but the license to begin learning. As Sir William Osler famously stated, 'The physician who winds up his work with his degree, and does not go on as a student, is to be pitied.'

"Education is not the filling of a pail, but the lighting of a fire."

— William Butler Yeats

1. Beyond the Lecture: The Mechanics of Self-Directed Learning (SDL)

SDL is a four-step process: identifying learning needs, setting goals, identifying resources, and evaluating outcomes. It is driven by the 'Clinical Gap'—the space between what a doctor knows and what they need to know to heal the patient in front of them.

CASE STUDY: THE PIVOT OF DR. ARIS

Dr. Aris, a seasoned GP, encountered a patient with refractory chronic pain not responding to standard protocols. Instead of defaulting to higher-dose opioids, he used the PICO framework to search for neuroplastic pain interventions. By actively seeking new knowledge, he integrated a new biopsychosocial modality into his entire practice. This is the essence of SDL: the patient is the ultimate curriculum.

2. The Art of Discernment: Critical Appraisal

Critical appraisal involves asking three questions: Are the results valid? What are the results? Will the results help me in caring for my patient? Lifelong learners must look beyond statistical significance (p-values) to clinical significance and Effect Size.

3. The Friday Curiosities: Creating a Culture of Inquiry

CASE STUDY: DR. PATEL'S CURIOSITY ROUNDS

Dr. Patel dedicated every Friday morning to 'curiosity rounds' to research rare conditions seen during the week. This ritual transformed his practice from transactional service into a social, celebratory 'Community of Practice.' Curiosity is the primary antidote to burnout.

4. Leveraging Technology: The Digital Physician

Professional development today involves curated 'Personal Learning Networks' (PLNs) and tools like FOAMed. Integration of AI is the next frontier, but tools must augment, rather than replace, critical thinking.

Practitioner Reflections

- What was the last clinical question you wrote down to research later?
- How many times did you say, 'I don't know, let's find out together'?
- How do you balance new evidence with clinical judgment?

References

Mann, K. V. (2011). Theoretical perspectives in medical education. Medical Education.

Sackett, D. L., et al. (1996). Evidence based medicine: what it is and what it isn't. BMJ.

Wenger, E. (1998). Communities of Practice: Learning, Meaning, and Identity.

Patel, R. (2020). The Curiosity Rounds: Reinvigorating the Clinician Scientist.

Chapter 14: Legal Aspects of Medical Practice: Understanding Liability and Risk Management

Learning Objectives

- Define the four elements of medical negligence and their practical implications.
- Differentiate between the legal requirements and the ethical spirit of informed consent.
- Develop advanced clinical documentation strategies that serve as a 'witness' in legal proceedings.
- Implement risk management protocols to mitigate errors and improve patient safety.
- Understand the psychological impact of litigation on the healthcare provider and the patient.

Practicing medicine is often likened to walking a tightrope. On one side lies the immense satisfaction of healing; on the other, the profound responsibility of human life. In the modern era, this tightrope is suspended over a complex legal landscape. For the clinical master, legal knowledge is not merely a tool for ' defensive medicine,' but a foundational pillar of professional excellence. As noted by Blackie (2021), 'The law does not require perfection, but it does require reasonableness, transparency, and a commitment to the standard of care.'

"The physician's best defence is not a clever lawyer, but a lifetime of thoroughness and empathy." — Anonymous

14.1 Negligence and Duty of Care

Medical malpractice or negligence is not simply a 'bad outcome.' It is a specific legal failure. To succeed in a claim, a plaintiff must establish four elements: Duty, Breach, Causation, and Damages (Bal, 2009).

Duty of Care: In the eyes of the law, a duty begins the moment a doctor-patient relationship is established. This requires acting according to the 'standard of care.'

Breach of Duty: Occurs when the clinician's conduct falls below the accepted standard.

Causation: The breach must be the 'but-for' cause of the injury.

Damages: There must be actual harm—physical, emotional, or financial.

Clinical Focus: Excellence in documentation is the best defence. In court, the prevailing maxim remains: 'If it isn't written down, it didn't happen.' Detailed, objective, and timely notes are clinical artifacts that prove a clinician's thought process.

14.2 Informed Consent: The Process vs. The Paper

Informed consent is a dynamic process of communication (Mabaso, 2022). A truly 'informed' patient understands three things: The nature and purpose of the procedure, the risks (even rare ones), and the viable alternatives.

Case Study: The Protective Power of Detail

Scenario: Dr. Sarah performed a complex spinal fusion. The patient developed a rare nerve palsy (<1% incidence) and sued. Outcome: The lawsuit was dropped because Dr. Sarah's notes included a handwritten diagram and a specific note detailing the conversation about the 1 in 1000 risk profile. Analysis: Detailed documentation of the conversation led the plaintiff's attorney to drop the case before trial.

14.3 Proactive Risk Management and Systems Thinking

Risk management requires moving from a 'Blame Culture' to a 'Safety Culture' (Reason, 2000). Key strategies include:

Structured (SBAR) communication to reduce miscommunication.

Incident Reporting to learn from 'near misses.'

Emotional Intelligence: Compassionate communication significantly reduces the likelihood of being sued (Levinson et al., 1997).

Chapter Reflections

1. Am I treating the legal record as a chore or as a clinical asset?
2. Do my patients feel heard, or like they are being processed through a machine?
3. How do I react when a colleague points out a potential error?

References

Bal, B. S. (2009). An introduction to medical malpractice in the United States. Clinical Orthopaedics.

Blackie, M. (2021). The Reasonable Physician: Standards of Care in Modern Law. Healthcare Press.

Levinson, W., et al. (1997). Physician-patient communication and malpractice claims. JAMA.

Mabaso, T. (2022). Ethics and the Law in African Healthcare. University Press.

Reason, J. (2000). Human error: models and management. BMJ.

Chapter 15: The Future of Excellence: Trends and Challenges in Healthcare

As we look toward the mid-21st century, the definition of excellence will evolve to meet new global challenges, from climate-related health issues to personalized genomics.

Personalized Medicine

The "one size fits all" approach to clinical practice is rapidly giving way to the era of precision medicine. In this new paradigm, treatments are no longer based solely on broad population averages but are meticulously tailored to the unique genetic profile, environment, and lifestyle of the individual. This shift promises to maximize therapeutic efficacy while minimizing adverse reactions, marking a pinnacle of medical excellence.

Global Health and Equity

Future excellence will be measured not just by the technological sophistication of our interventions, but by our ability to deliver care to the most vulnerable populations globally. True medical leadership in the coming decades will involve bridging the health equity gap, ensuring that life-saving innovations are accessible to all, regardless of geographic location or socio-economic status.

CASE STUDY: THE AI EVOLUTION

"The rise of AI-driven diagnostics suggests a future where the physician's role shifts from a 'repository of facts' to a 'curator of wisdom and compassion.'"

As artificial intelligence takes over the heavy lifting of data synthesis and pattern recognition, the human element of medicine becomes more critical than ever. Excellence in the future will be defined by the physician's ability to navigate complex ethical landscapes and provide the empathetic guidance that machines cannot replicate.

Don't miss out!

Visit the website below and you can sign up to receive emails whenever Mbuso Mabuza publishes a new book. There's no charge and no obligation.

https://books2read.com/r/B-A-JPJL-OKBZI

BOOKS 2 READ

Connecting independent readers to independent writers.

Did you love *Excellence In Medicine*? Then you should read *Promoting Health and Wellbeing*[1] by Mbuso Mabuza!

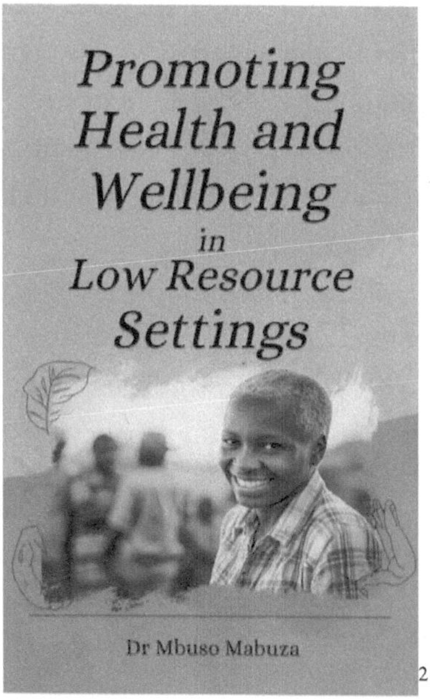

[2]

Promoting Health and Wellbeing in Low Resource Settings offers a transformative perspective on public health, moving beyond traditional disease prevention to address health as a multifaceted societal effort. This essential guide bridges the gap between theory and action, providing a roadmap for navigating the complexities of health promotion where resources are limited but the potential for impact is limitless.

· Core Insights & Strategic Themes

Evolution of Health: Understand health as a result of social, political, and economic environments rather than just medical outcomes.

---

1. https://books2read.com/u/bPgYrR

2. https://books2read.com/u/bPgYrR

Global Impact: Navigate shifting international trends and their direct influence on local communities.

Community Empowerment: Master participatory approaches and strategies to work directly with people for sustainable change.

Advocacy & Policy: Gain expertise in leveraging public policy and mass media to reshape community health narratives.

Practical Application: Follow step-by-step guidance on needs assessment, program development, and rigorous evaluation.

An Indispensable Resource

Whether you are a clinician, policymaker, community leader, or student, this book equips you with evidence-based strategies to foster empowerment. It is the definitive toolkit for the next generation of practitioners dedicated to improving quality of life in marginalized communities worldwide.

Also by Mbuso Mabuza

A Healthy Mind And Best You: Achieving Great Results in Every Aspect of Your Life
Purposeful And Better You
Efficacy, Effectiveness And Efficiency In The Management Of Health Systems
Promoting Health and Wellbeing
Medicine and the Sociology of Health
Qualitative Methods In Public Health Research
Global Health Disaster Management
Global Health Policy And Programme Challenges
The Journey of Life Has a Gift of Purpose
Epidemiological Research
Ethics, Qualitative And Quantitative Methods In Public Health Research
Emotional Intelligence in Relationships
Blockchain Technology In Healthcare And Medicine
Immersive Technologies In Healthcare: Virtual Reality And Augmented Reality
Health Data Analytics And Informatics
How To Improve The Way You Think
Health Systems Engineering: Building A Better Healthcare Delivery System
Artificial Intelligence In Drug Discovery And Development
How To Make The Most Of Life
Precision Medicine

Connected Health: Technology-Enabled Care
Person Centered Care And Optimal Wellbeing
Reimagine Your Tomorrow
Leading Remote Teams in the 21st Century
Qualitative Research In Health and Medicine
Excellence In Medicine

About the Author

Dr. Mbuso Mabuza is a distinguished leader with over 20 years of experience across the global health and public service sectors. He has held influential roles at *Johns Hopkins Bloomberg School of Public Health*, *The World Bank*, and *Transnet*, managing complex health portfolios and strategic initiatives.

Currently a prominent academic, Dr. Mabuza focuses on bridging the gap between practical leadership and academic excellence. His expertise uniquely intersects policy, health management, and clinical practice to drive sustainable global impact.

Read more at drmbusomabuzabooks.com.

www.ingramcontent.com/pod-product-compliance
Lightning Source LLC
LaVergne TN
LVHW101617210926
848480LV00009B/735

* 9 7 9 8 2 3 3 9 8 8 8 2 0 *